THE ITCH and What to Do Besides Scratching

J. I. Rodale

RODALE BOOKS, INC., EMMAUS, PENNA. 18049

Standard Book Number 87596-049-9

Printed in the United States
G-718
First Printing—March, 1971

Table of Contents

Chapter 1.

TORTURE SHORT OF PAIN

"Where are you going?"

"I'm going to get a dollar's worth of scratch-paper."

"But that'll last you for years!"

"I know it. I've got the seven-year itch."

This is a popular joke . . . but a very old one, as you can see from the use of the expression "scratch-paper," which no doubt means sandpaper. The mere mention of the word "itch" on the stage always brings a laugh. This has been true right down through the ages. Even Socrates joked about the pleasures of itching and scratching. Yet, this could be a very serious and painful condition, and millions of dollars are spent each year for remedies to relieve it. At one time or another in life it affects almost all persons.

In the time of Henry VIII the scabies

was so common in England that it was called "The English Itch." When people wore wigs they became infected with lice, which encouraged scratching. King Louis XIV had a small room issuing off the great Hall of Mirrors where he would go to change wigs, when the one he wore became too "active." People must have scratched regularly in those days. This was especially true about the Chinese, who developed back-scratchers carved in the shape of a hand, which were standard equipment in all houses.

Samuel Pepys, in his diary for the day of January 23, 1669, says:

"So to my wife's chamber, and there supped, and got her to cut my hair and look at my shirt, for I have itched mightily these six or seven days, and when it all comes to all she finds that I am lousy, having found in my head and body about 20 lice, little and great, which I wonder at, being more than I have had these 20 years. I did think I might have got them from the little boy, but they did presently look at him, and found none. So how they come I know not, but presently did shift myself, and so shall be rid of them, and cut my hair close to my head, and so with much content to bed."

In those days daily bathing was not as common as it is today. The bathing facilities were so crude that it took a bit of doing to give oneself a decent washing. So we might put down the first fact that we have learned about how to prevent itching which is, that if you will bathe more you will itch less, although, sometimes the itch is more deep-seated than that, as we shall see.

In medical discussions and articles the term *pruritus* is used to indicate itching. To show the low status of the word, a similar-sounding word, *prurience,* means lewdness in thought or desire. An "itch plant," which is found in tropical countries and which is used to make itching powder, is called *mucuna pruriens.* According to some medical opinion, scratching an itch is a form of masturbation, although this idea is pooh-poohed by most physicians.

Why do people scratch? Some believe that the pain produced by the scratching is a means of stopping the itching. The physiological explanation is that itching stops when pain supervenes. But the explanation lies deeper. Scratching causes a quicker circulation of the blood, thus acting to eliminate, perhaps temporarily, the condition that has caused the itch. If people could improve the circulation of their blood by daily exercise and other good health practices, there would be less itching. So now we have two preventives: frequent bathing and sufficient exercise.

A great amount of research has been done in this field, but people continue to scratch. The doctors have even gone so far as to develop a scratching machine that is used in research to study the effect of the friction of scratching on the skin. They want to find out how much scratching will produce that raw, leathery appearance of the skin called lichenification. The machine tests the strength of the epidermis, and it has been found that after a certain amount of friction has been applied the epidermis suddenly will give way. Well and good, but more time should be spent on what man can do to prevent the itching from occurring in the first place. Then we wouldn't scratch, and there would be no need for scratching machines.

Scratching is a reflex action to itching. Itch . . . scratch! "That's all there is to it," you think? Not so with the psychiatrists. They don't think that way at all. To a psychiatrist scratching may provide a satisfaction for thwarted desires or self-punishment for guilty thoughts or deeds. This opinion is almost as bad as that of the masturbation school, isn't it?

What is an itch? It has been defined as a form of pain. As one doctor has expressed it, "Stimuli not sufficient to produce pain often gives rise to itching," or expressed another way, itching is a modified form of pain. It has also been called a deranged form of pain and pain gone wrong. But whatever it is, or has been called, it can be torture to a sensitive patient. Sometimes the itching is so bad that one would gladly trade it for pain. In some cases it is so severe that it leads to suicide.

Most frequently the itching occurs in the perianal area; that is, the midregion around the upper thighs and anus, front and back, including the area of the sexual organs. It is often worse at night; that is, in bed. In fact, in many cases the itching occurs only at this time. It could be that at such a time the circulation is at a lower ebb. All the body processes are moderated. Such a slowing down furnishes an excellent climate for places in the body to begin to itch. Stagnation of blood flow is a prominent cause of itching. That is why it so often occurs at the feet, a point so far away from the heart that its power to pump blood there is somewhat reduced, especially in cases of heart disease and other circulatory conditions.

Itching is a symptom, not a disease in itself, but it always arises because a disease condition is beginning to develop. Thus, itching has an informative function. It is a signal that damage is occurring somewhere in the body, and therefore it has real clinical significance. A routine question asked by doctors should be, not "Do you itch anywhere?" but "Where do you itch?"

As has been said, itching is a common symptom of disease, after certain local conditions are ruled out such as senile skin, sunburn, bath itch, winter itch, insect bites, etc. It could stem from practically any disease, which is a reason why it comes under the sphere of the surgeon, the gynecologist who deals with genitourinary and rectal diseases of women, the proctologist who specializes on the rectum and its diseases, the dermatologist, allergist, psychiatrist, or what have you. This is the reason why patients in torment go from practitioner to practitioner, from specialist to specialist.

Everything is tried short of dynamite. In fact, in desperation some physicians have resorted to tattooing the affected part, as this is supposed to give relief. Do they tattoo pictures of St. Vitus?

And, as is only human, many specialists believe . . . they are absolutely certain in fact . . . that the particular itch you have comes within their specialty and that their disease speciality is the cause of the pruritus. The allergist believes it is due to an allergy, the dermatologist that it is a disease of the skin, and the psychiatrist that you hate your mother-in-law. As one physician so aptly put it, "In our experience, some of the worst treatment failures occurred after months of therapy by a stubborn specialist who would not recognize the importance of other possible causes."

Sometimes the doctor doesn't think it a good thing to cure the pruritus too fast. I will quote a statement made by George M. Lewis, M.D., (*N.Y. Journal of Medicine,* May 15, 1957):

"Itch is sometimes not bad for a patient. That may seem rather heartless but we know that if you cure pruritus ani (itching rectum) abruptly, the patient may proceed to acquire some other condition, perhaps one that is worse or harder to handle. Just dwelling on that thought for a moment, we might say then that using hydrocortisone ointment, which is to me almost a miracle drug in this location, is perhaps not the best kind of treatment. Perhaps we should get the patient only slightly or mostly better but not completely well, allowing him to have some symptom which may be an emotional outlet. I am not a psychiatrist but I believe we all have to use psychiatric skills in the treatment of pruritus ani."

Personally, I would rather get completely cured of the itch, if I had it, and find some other emotional outlet.

Bathe often!

Get plenty of exercise!

Be healthy! This means, follow the *Prevention* system of good nutrition.

Don't get into such trouble that it will affect your spirit!

And don't scratch!

Chapter 2.

FOODS THAT CAUSE ITCHING

Before we go into a full discussion in connection with the various causes of the itch, or pruritus, it might be best first to consider a most common cause of self-inflicted itching, usually of the anal or rectum region, and that is the food we eat. In some cases the cause may be allergy, in others it may be directly produced by some deleterious compound in the food.

You wouldn't think that sugar could be a cause of pruritus ani (itchy rectum). Here is a letter recently received from Miss W. R. Fink of Marshall, Michigan, regarding this complaint:

"I have been suffering from this ailment since I was a young girl. Doctors have not been able to help me. Friends have advised me to stop eating tomatoes and strawberries, as they thought it might be the acid these contain which caused the difficulty. I found no great improvement by following this advice.

"However, about two years ago, I had some tomatoes in my garden which I ate, and the itching grew very bad. Then I recalled that I had read a lot about refined white *sugar* being bad for you. I had always eaten fruits and tomatoes with *sugar*. I decided to omit the *sugar*, and of all the surprises I ever had this was the greatest! I got better instead of worse. Since then nobody can give me anything that has white *sugar* in it. I use a little brown *sugar* —not more than five pounds a year and I have got the pruritus ani whipped. I am 86 years old and now after an ulcerated colon and cancerous tumor removed, I cannot thank God and *Prevention* enough for being able to enjoy the best of health."

A physician, F. B. Bowman, M.D., in a letter to *The Canadian Medical Association Journal*, Sept. 1, 1955, indicts the cola drinks as a cause of pruritus ani, and it probably is the sugar in them that is the culprit. He says, "*Chocolate*, in my experience, is one of the most frequent offenders. *Peanut butter* and *peanuts*, and *honey*, are a few of the most common irritants. A young nurse who was addicted to *cola drinks* was in misery, and had to discontinue her course in training. When she stopped drinking six to eight bottles of it a day, the condition cleared up." He winds up by stating that pruritus ani is not a case for the dermatologist, but should be handled by the proctologist. A proctologist is a physician who deals with diseases of the rectum and anus.

This same Dr. Bowman took part in a discussion on pruritus ani which was reported in the November, 1951, issue of *The American Journal of Surgery* in which he said, "I have found that 3 or 4 foods are frequently the culprits. Inquiry is made as to whether *chocolate*, *peanut butter*, *margarine* or *honey* is used. The question is asked, always, 'Are you a *cola* drinker?' I think of a doctor who consulted me in such a state that he was considering giving up practice. On questioning him, I found that he was a confirmed *chocolate* eater. The condition was as bad or worse than any discussed by the speaker. In a very short time he was perfectly well after stopping his *chocolate*. If he takes an ABS and C coated laxative tablet it will throw him into a spasm of pruritus ani."

Another physician, commenting on what Dr. Bowman said, stated, "Dr. Bowman was dead right in thinking of the diets, allergies and all that group. That is terribly important and, as he mentioned, *chocolate* is one of the greatest offenders in the whole group and will cause pruritus. Restriction of it will help. The greatest offender of all is *alcohol*. I have had people test themselves to see how quickly *alcohol* had an effect. They said within a few hours, and certainly by the next morning the pruritus was back again. The only way I can figure *alcohol* works is that it must work through its stimulation of the central nervous system and in turn be related to this emotional disturbance."

A doctor writes to *Modern Medicine*, October 1, 1955, issue, describes the case of a 75-year old male patient who has severe pruritus ani after eating *beef*, and asks for advice. Have the patient stop eating *beef*, replied the editor. This, he said, was the only solution he knew. I imagine that *beef* would be a rare kind of food to cause *pruritus*, but evidently it does sometimes.

Wheat products have been found to cause itching anus where the latter is due to celiac disease. In the adult form this condition is known as steatorrhea, which is a condition of fat in the stools. There is also irritability, abdominal distension and pruritus ani. Staying away from all gluten-containing products, such as *wheat*, *rye*, etc., results in a clearing up of all these symptoms. The disease and the itch are caused by these *bread* foods and are cured by their elimination.

In my own case I have found *citrus* fruit and *pineapple* to be a cause of pruritus ani. The other day I ate a half a slice of *pineapple*, and there was the pruritus, the very next morning. By far the greatest villain of them all is *citrus* fruit. I used to suffer fearfully by reason of it until a pharmacist told me what trouble drinking orange juice could cause in the rectal region. He proved this to his own satisfaction any number of times. I immediately cut out all forms of *citrus,* namely orange, grapefruit and lemon, and my troubles were over. I mentioned this to a friend of mine who suffered from pruritus ani, and he also cut out *citrus* fruit from his diet. Within a few days he was relieved of all itching.

A reader from Colorado wrote us that a rectal operation had left him with a painful and distressing case of pruritus ani. Doctors suggested a number of salves, none of which helped him in the slightest. Then they suggested x-ray treatments. After reading *Prevention,* this reader decided instead to stop eating *citrus* fruit. "In a week the itching stopped," he wrote. "It is a bit tender and sensitive, but I have not been bothered by the itching for more than 3 months."

Here is a letter from Lizabeth Wiley of Greybull, Wyoming: "I found some very useful information in *Prevention,* a letter signed by a man who stated he had cured himself of intense itching in the rectum by discontinuing the use of *citrus* fruits. I had a very severe case of itching in the rectum, mouth of bladder and exterior parts; also a breaking out of a rash that caused intense itching externally as well as internally. I thought the man's treatment worth trying. I quit *citrus* fruit, and in little more than a week all itching was gone, and it has not returned. I eat an orange occasionally; sometimes half a grapefruit. I had been in a reputable clinic for consultation and examination, but they found no remedy. I saw the latter in *Prevention* and soon found the cure."

In an article in the May 15, 1952, issue of *Modern Medicine* covering pruritus ani, Neil W. Swinton, M.D., of the Lahey Clinic, Boston, said that excessive *carbohydrate* intake increases the alkalinity of the rectal region, which is one of the causes of itching. In this respect he also says, "Excessive *fruit juices* in the diet and alcohol may be significant at times." In another article in *Modern Medicine*, July 15, 1957, appears the statement, "Foods and drinks that may irritate the involved area include excessive *citrus* fruits or juices, *condiments*, strong *alcoholic beverages*, *nuts* and *popcorn*."

According to an item in the *Southern*

Medical Journal for October, 1949, F. R. Rugeley, M.D., reveals that the following foods have caused pruritus ani. The number in front of each food indicates the number of times he came across this particular allergy in his practice. 7—wheat, 3—eggs, 3—beef, 3—milk, 2—figs, 2—tomatoes, 1—asparagus, 1—dewberry, 1—white potato, 1—sweet potato, 1—beans.

Some opinion has it that what causes the trouble is drinking orange juice from unripe oranges. California oranges, for example, are usually picked green. To me the offending element in the citrus is the citric acid, a very powerful substance, and it matters not whether it is in green or ripe oranges. However, tests can be made to determine the accuracy of that opinion. The citric acid does a great deal of harm in many ways other than in causing pruritus. In past issues of *Prevention,* and in our *Health Finder* and *Health Builder,* we have shown the following troublesome conditions that have resulted from overconsumption of citrus fruits: tooth erosion, headaches, physical exhaustion, stomach pains, dizziness, prolonged colds, joint pains, sinusitis, bleeding gums, loss of weight, digestive disorders, cramps, rash, infected fingernails.

If you are concerned over the fact that by eliminating citrus you will not be getting sufficient vitamin C, you can be assured of a liberal amount of it by taking rose hip tablets. Food rich in vitamin C are tomatoes, green peppers, broccoli, brussel sprouts, cabbage, cantaloup, etc.

We have seen that the following foods can cause pruritus ani in some cases:

Sugar	Asparagus
Chocolate	Dewberry
Peanut Butter	Potatoes
Peanuts	Beans
Honey	Beef
Cola Drinks	Wheat, rye, etc.
Margarine	Pineapple
Alcohol	Citrus
Eggs	Condiments
Milk	Nuts
Figs	Popcorn
Tomatoes	Excess carbohydrates

As you look at this list you must understand that there are two different principles involved in their use . . . an allergy to food or, secondly, a direct chemical effect because of some offending element in the food. As far as allergy is concerned, almost any food could cause it in some persons, because there is something wrong with these persons.

According to medical opinion, their body forms a compound called histamine which disrupts body cells, injuring the small capillaries through which serum will ooze, causing hives (swelling of the skin), watering eyes and nose, etc. If it affects the lungs, it causes asthma. But, if such an allergic person becomes health-conscious, especially if he follows the complete *Prevention* system, he can gradually do away with his allergies, as I have. For example, years ago the eating of onion would raise my pulse, which is a symptom of allergy. Today I can eat all the onion I want.

Now in the second category, such as citrus and bread, there are compounds in it (citric acid in citrus) which exert a direct harmful effect in most everyone, and the only thing one can do is to eliminate such foods, or consume them in extreme moderation. In allergies there is no such thing as moderation. A crumb or a drop of the offender is enough to produce symptoms.

In the case of allergies, one must check for oneself by a process of elimination and the use of the Coca system of checking the pulse after consuming each item of food in one's diet. See our *Health Finder*. By careful observation and experience one can usually eliminate any itch that is caused by food, merely by the elimination of that food.

Chapter 3.

SKIN IS SENSITIVE

There are a thousand causes underlying a condition of itching. They can include anything from dandruff to diabetes. There was the case of the minister who developed an inconvenient itch on his palms. He had a habit of looking out of his window, resting his palms on the painted windowsill. Evidently there was something in the paint that irritated his skin. Itchy palm of a theatre cashier was caused by contact with the metal counter of her ticket vending machine. In one case itching was tracked down to the blue dye in the yarn that a woman was using for her knitting.

Much pruritus today is caused by the thousands of new chemical compounds used in articles we employ every day, in such products as plastics, cosmetics, disinfectants, detergents, antiseptics, fabrics, drugs, deodorants, soaps, body lotions, underwear, douches, contraceptives, colored toilet paper, nail polish, etc. One physician sums up the list of local causes as "animal parasites, local secretions, disease, heat or cold, chemical irritants, vegetable irritants such as nettles or fungi, and mechanical irritants such as scratching and rubbing, the rubbing of clothing and the effect of the wind."

There are all kinds of special itches such as barber's itch, farmer's itch, miner's, swimmer's, lumberman's, grocer's, baker's, harvest, copra, water, onion, grain, barley, and winter itch. But in all such cases there is always some offending element that can be tracked down with a little trouble. For example, winter itch may be due to an intolerance of winter underwear.

Excessive use of soap is a common source of itching. Ultraviolet lamps have caused the hands to break out. People on extremely low fat diets have suffered moderately. A 63 year old man developed pruritus of the face and eyelids from "Thermofax" duplicating paper. There is nylon stockings dermatitis, which is caused by a certain kind of dye (AZO) used in them. Pure nylon does not cause it. It may be caused also by nylon hairnets. In this case it is a sensitivity to the resin finish in which the net is coated.

Shoemakers get a form of eczema, which itches severely, from a new kind of glue which contains a phenolformaldehyde synthetic resin. Woolen and other rough-textured clothing may be an aggravating factor in itching. A woman working with fiberglass in a factory suffered an eruption of fingers, hands, forearms and wrists, and it was so bad she had to be hospitalized. Discontinuing this job effected a complete cure. It was found that it was not the fiberglass that brought about the eruption. Again it was a phenol-formaldehyde synthetic resin that was used as a bonding substance in the fiberglass.

A doctor reports a case of a woman who developed a troublesome pruritus in the anal region. She had believed it was caused by hemorrhoids, and treated herself with suppositories and salves, which only caused the itching to increase. It was finally discovered that menthol in the salves was an irritating factor. She had an eczema which originated from sensitization with menthol as a result of its chronic use.

Many persons are sensitive to nickel contained in such articles as hair grips, spectacles, earrings, necklaces, brooches, pins, brassieres, zip-fasteners, suspenders, corsets, scissors, watches, bracelets, shoe buckles, etc. Here's a typical case from the *British Medical Journal* (June 23, 1956):

"With reference to nickel sensitivity, may I quote one case which I hope will be of interest to fellow practitioners? A young woman, aged 17, came to see me, complaining of a rash on her chest which was obviously caused by the metal brassiere clips she was wearing. Treatment was given, and she was warned against wearing nickel close to her skin. She was not seen again for eight months. Reappearing after that interval, a papulovesicular rash was noted on her face and neck, with oedema of the eyelids (three days' duration). Similar lesions were present on the flexures of her arms and on the thighs, yet on careful examination no primary lesion was detectable at that time. On interrogation she admitted buying a pair of metal suspenders, but had worn them less than one week. Forty hours later a large patch of dermatitis appeared behind her left thigh."

Itching and scratching by factory employees cost U.S. Industry more than a hundred million ($100,000,000) dollars a year. These conditions are usually caused by chemical compounds that the workers handle. There are newer and more powerful chemicals being developed and the company doctors must keep ever on the lookout because of them. A typical example is butyraldoxime, a printing ink chemical, which causes pruritus in printers after they drink alcoholic beverages. Plant sanitation, air-conditioning, protective clothing such as special types of aprons, helmets and gloves, showering before going home are preventive measures.

A great many men itch between the thighs, and this may be due to perspiration caused by tight and heavy trousers and underwear at that point. Scotchmen who wear kilts do not have this affliction. Men who do a lot of sitting should try to keep their legs spread apart so as to allow free ventilation of the thighs. Clothing should be light and woolen garments should not be in contact with the skin. People should be careful not to cross their legs when sitting because it creates a wet perspiredness between the thighs, a condition which allows fungi to breed there and cause pruritus. Besides, the pressure of one leg pressing upon another impedes the blood circulation, which does not make for a healthy skin.

I have often wondered why a person sometimes itches more in the night than in the daytime. It could be that in bed the warmth of the covering causes perspiration which remains on the skin for the duration of the night.

A common cause of pruritus is an unhealthy skin. The part that nutrition plays in it will be discussed later, but here we will discuss other aspects of keeping the skin in good condition. Cleanliness is important, but overbathing can lead to trouble. Too frequent hot baths will cause itching because they remove natural oil from the skin, leaving it too dry. Some people put a couple of tablespoonfuls of salad oil in the bath. Old people suffer from dry skin which is an accompaniment of old age. Because of this they should lubricate their skin with olive oil. The following is a medical suggestion as to a special kind of bath that aids a dry old skin. A cup of starch, bran or oatmeal is shaken in a quart milk bottle with two tablespoonfuls of lubricating oil and then thoroughly mixed with a quart of milk and poured into half a tubful of lukewarm water. Avoid the use of soap, or at least limit its use to underarms and the thighs. Much trouble is caused by soap, and I haven't used it for years, except in the thigh region. I use the wash rag vigorously.

The Medical Press of London has a few words to say on this subject:

"The skin in this area also appears to be extremely sensitive, not only to certain soaps, contraceptives and antiseptic douches, but also to lotions, ointments, fungicides and medicated pessaries, especially those containing tar, cocaine derivatives, sulphonamides, penicillin and arsenic. It may happen, therefore, that a woman who is meticulous in her cleanliness may develop pruritus from local skin sensitivity (contact dermatitis) to the agents employed, and that remedies prescribed by her doctor may do more harm than good."

A lack of good circulation will contribute to a poor skin and cause itching. Exercise is indicated in such a case, and body massage.

It is important to have a healthy skin. Sugars in artificial form contribute to skin disease. The rich custards, cakes, pies, ice cream sodas, sugary sweets, and starches provide fertile soil for the growth of bacteria in the skin, and make one more susceptible to skin infections. If there is a constant history of pruritus, the sweet tooth should be curbed.

A patient with generalized itching, without a skin rash, may have a disease such as diabetes, a tumor, jaundice, Hodgkin's disease, or leukemia, and in many cases itching is associated with the change of life (menopause). Diabetes is a very common cause and itching then affects the obese diabetic especially. Itching may also be caused by measles, scarlet fever, liver and gall bladder disease, blood disorders, nephritis, gastritis, dyspepsia and sexual disturbances in the female. It is, therefore, important, if one of these diseases is the cause, that it be properly diagnosed and treated.

The use of the antibiotic drugs has been found to cause itching and burning of the anus, but sometimes it takes 4 to 8 weeks for the result of these to show itself, and by that time the origin is forgotten. Aureomycin especially is a common offender. The itching is so intense that scaly encrustations and excoriations appear because of violent scratching. Many other drugs cause pruritus. Examples are nupercainal, chloramphenicol, and mecamylamine.

Now we come to the psychosomatic aspects of the subject. "As with love, it is difficult to know where it is bred, in the skin or in the head." The mind can affect the skin. As an example, fear can bring about goose-flesh. Nervous tension can cause perspiration of the feet which could trigger an attack of athlete's foot. That the pruritus is sometimes in the mind can be seen in the case where the foot that has been amputated still itches. A lot of trouble is caused by stubborn dermatologists who keep on treating the patient, ignoring completely the psychosomatic possibilities.

The Medical Press (Feb. 22, 1958) says, "There are several reasons why emotional disturbances affect the skin more than most other organs. The skin is the chief organ of emotional expression. Across its surface flit the flush of anger or excitement, the blush of shame or confusion, the pallor and cold sweat of fear, the goose-flesh of terror, and the itch of frustrated 'drives' or longings . . . The skin is exposed more than any other organ to physical and chemical damage and to infections. Anxiety may cause itching and this may set off a chain reaction of pathological processes in the skin."

Dermatologists have coined a word for the ailment of people who only think they have an itch. They call this condition *acarophobia*. Various emotions such as insecurity, anxiety, worry, hostility, guilt, frustration, family maladjustments, depression, financial upsets, feelings of resentment, hatred, sexual maladjustment and generally unpleasant situations can cause upsets in the nervous system that lead to flushing, sweating and itching. But when the patient learns what is at the bottom of his condition, he is on the way towards a cure.

Quoted in *Science News Letter* (Dec. 17, 1949) Dr. Frank E. Cornia of New York City says that patients and others "who suffer intense itching or burning sensations in just one or two spots are unconsciously haboring feelings of resentment or hatred toward a close relative or toward their work, which may be unsuitable to them." In a study of 300 patients, Dr. Cornia found that more than half, 57%, had severe disturbances in their family situation. Maladjustments in early life affected 77%, and long-standing conflicts in adult life affected as many as 87%. Abnormal strictness of parents, family strife, sexual difficulties and unsuitable work actually caused the severe itching and skin disturbances.

Here are several cases described in the

British Journal of Dermatology (64: 274-280, 1952): "Resentment may be outstanding. In one case a mother, upset by noisy children and a jealous husband, concealed her reactions but itched when agitated. The patient improved when encouraged to express herself freely. A little girl cooped up with intolerant grandparents was not helped by treatment."

In another case severe itching was thought to be caused in a young man by the tensions of his honeymoon, but when it was thoroughly investigated it was found that the condition was caused by contact sensitivity of the patient's skin to the perfumes and cosmetics his wife was using, which shows that we must keep our wits about us in dealing with the problem of pruritus.

CHAPTER 4.

PRURITUS ANI

In a previous section we went into the causes of itching generally, including pruritus ani (itching rectum). Here we shall limit ourselves exclusively to pruritus ani. According to one physician (*Medical Journal of Australia*, 4/26/58), "Pruritus ani is frequently the only symptom and ofttimes it occurs in the absence of any physical sign. It is more common in men than in women, in the elderly than in the young, in summer than in winter, and in neurotics than in psychotics. It may be acute or chronic, and it waxes and wanes." A psychotic is a person characterized by a deep, far-reaching and prolonged behavior disorder.

In reference to the statement above that pruritus ani affects men more often than women certain doctors (Weiss and English) in 1957 claimed that in their experience all female patients suffering from

P.A. were frigid. This statement is questioned by other physicians. Some psychiatrists claim that P.A. is always an indication of latent or overt homosexual tendencies. This is such an exaggeration that it isn't even funny. Some physicians admit that in *some* cases there may be something amiss in the patient's sexual relationship . . . sexual perversion or a lack of gratification, but such cases are rare.

For the most part P.A. is caused by allergies, or can be due to certain diseases, or to various foods, and can also be psychosomatic. Many authorities have also ascribed it to a state of vitamin-deficiency. The reason it shows itself in the anal region is that the skin is highly sensitive there. There is also a moisture, which is not very helpful.

A disorder in a person's metabolism can produce it. Diseases like jaundice, diabetes, gout and pregnancy can be responsible for it. Drugs, laxatives and the antibiotics can bring it about. Excess alcohol, tobacco, or highly seasoned food can be causes of it.

Listed among other causes are newsprint, x-rays, lack of cleanliness, excess washing, leakage of mucus through the anus, senility, tumors, leakage of liquid paraffin (mineral oil) through the anus, threadworms, fungus infections, and you might say a thousand other things. If you have it, you or your doctor must be a detective and track down the cause. Remove it and the pruritus ceases. The cures are usually dramatic and self-satisfying.

In one study of pruritus ani (*The Journal of Investigative Dermatology*, June, 1941), 38 patients were studied. Some of them had suffered from P.A. for 20 years, although the average period was 2 years. After investigating for allergies that could have caused the pruritus, the doctors found the following to be the offending things:

Patient A:

Rabbit, potato, dog, wheat, string beans, ascaris, cow, cherry. Wool, pyrethrum, almond, dust, chocolate, goat, rye, silkworm. Ragweed. plantain, timothy, trees.

Patient B:

Dust, ascaris, goat, timothy, silk, wool, ragweed, cow.

Patient C:

Wool, coffee, silkworm, dust, trees, tobacco, goat, ascaris, dog, pyrethrum, feathers.

Patient D:

Dust, pyrethrum, cow, wool, tobacco, goat, plantain, wheat, rye, rice.

Patient E:

Wheat, milk, chocolate, mustard, potato, orris, cat, rabbit, ascaris, ragweed, wool, dust, dog, pyrethrum, string beans.

Patient F:

Dust, wool, corn, silkworm, goat, feathers, coffee.

Patient G:

Wool, milk, dust, wheat.

Patient H:

Ascaris, feathers, rice, lamb, cabbage, peas, beans.

Patient I:

Silkworm, cow, wheat, rice, corn, wool, dust, glue.

Patient K:

Wool, dust, flaxseed, wheat, rice, corn, silkworm, buckwheat, lima beans.

Patient L:

Ragweed, dust, flaxseed, chocolate, almond, wheat, silk, wool, milk.

But in only 6 of the 38 patients with P.A. was a cure effected. This is an extremely poor batting average. I am amazed that the citrus fruits were not found as an offending agent. The drinking of orange juice is so common that it should always be suspected. But the trouble is that I do not believe its use reflects itself as an allergy. I believe it is purely a strong chemical irritant, some of the citric acid leaking out through the anus. When oranges are consumed whole, it is possible that the presence of pulp aids in more efficient absorption of all parts of the fruit.

The overuse of citrus does not only cause itching rectum. Last week a woman told my wife that some years ago, being unable to conceive, she was advised to drink orange juice at every meal. In a few weeks there broke out a heavy rash on her breasts. It sometimes takes a month or more to show its effect.

There is an interesting article in re pruritus ani in the *American Journal of Digestive Diseases* (June, 1947). I shall let the doctor who wrote it speak for himself. "In 1941 I began swallowing large amounts of cotton fiber as a non-nutritive substitute for food to make food restriction or fasting easier. The fiber (surgical cotton cut up or chopped up so as to reduce its tendency to mat) was hard to swallow without suitable flavoring and I found no entirely satisfactory non-nutritive flavor. Hence, I generally swallowed the fiber after soaking it in orange juice or some other fruit juice. This, without other food, served to satisfy me during periods of about 3 days after which more nourishing food seemed to be needed and was eaten during one or two days. Then I would again return to the exclusive use of cotton fiber soaked in fruit juice. This regimen of alternately restricting and liberalizing my food intake appeared to be highly beneficial, but it became complicated by the development of intolerable anal pruritus and therefore had to be abandoned.

"The diet of cotton fiber and fruit juice was obviously responsible for the pruritus as the anal itching disappeared intermittently with the eating of more normal food and it also did not occur when the cotton fiber was swallowed after it was soaked in olive oil or when it was taken mixed with tapioca jelly or other food."

He says that the diet of cotton fiber and fruit juice was obviously responsible for the pruritus, not realizing that it was the orange juice that was the offender, for when the cotton was taken with olive oil, the pruritus did not occur. Many physicians do not seem to be aware that citrus juice is one of the principal causes of pruritus ani.

The doctor continues, "Later, paroxysmal itching (as if an insect were biting) occurred after the apparent mere passage of small amounts of gas."

In passing, I certainly would question the dangerous practice of using cotton fiber as a means of curbing the appetite, not only because it is a non-food and could shock the processes of digestion, but also because it has gone through a disinfectant process and contains residues of toxic disinfectants. In his article the doctor states, "In fact, my sanity was questioned in some medical quarters because of my use of cotton fiber and other non-nutritive materials." Enough said.

In a textbook entirely devoted to the rectum by H. E. Bacon (J. B. Lippincott), the following is given in reference to pruritus ani:

I. Predisposing Causes:
   - (a) Mental (worry, overwork, etc.).
   - (b) Habits (alcoholism, sedentary life).
   - (c) Constitutional (diabetes, gout, liver diseases, etc.).

II. Indirect Causes:

(a) Mechanical causes (fissures, fistula, hemorrhoids, etc.).

(b) Infection (cryptitis, lice, worms, scabies, fungi).

(c) Food sensitivity (tomatoes, berries, shellfish, etc.).

(d) Drugs (quinine, morphine, belladonna, etc.).

III. Direct Causes:

(a) Traumatic (abrasions, chafing, prolapsing hemorrhoids).

(b) Chemical (discharges from anal or vaginal regions).

(c) Skin diseases (eczema, scabies, fungus disease).

(d) Physical uncleanliness, excessive sweating.

He mentions food sensitivity such as that caused by tomatoes, berries, shellfish, but says not a word about the citrus. The reason may be that food sensitivity is determined by allergic scratch tests, but the citrus, not being an allergy-caused irritant would not show up in a scratch test. Its action is purely chemical, and is caused by the citric acid in the fruit.

In reviewing many articles on the allergic causes of pruritus ani, over and over again, I see the disregard of citrus as a factor. For example, there is a long article by Dr. F. R. Rugeley in *Annals of Allergy* (Sept.-Oct., 1946) presenting 14 cases of pruritus ani, in which many allergic foods were found that caused the pruritus. They included fish, avocado, pork, beef, wheat, prunes, apples, green peas, dewberries, potatoes, beets, yeast, chocolate, onions, string beans, rice, spinach, egg, . . . but you can see . . . no citrus, the only possible reason being that citrus acts chemically, and not as an allergy. In other words, it would not show up as an allergy by the needle-scratch method.

Sometimes constipation can cause pruritus ani. Dr. R. H. Aldrich in *Industrial Medicine* (Oct., 1943) says, "The constipation following starvation diets, plus the aversion most elderly females have toward drinking water, brings about a definite trauma (damage) to the anus by the passing of concrete-like stools.

"Among the direct causes, skin diseases especially fungus infections and intertrigo (a chafed patch of skin) must be considered of importance. Baird points out that the perianal region with its furrows and ridges is a definite inter-trigous surface, and an area in which fungi infection is the primary cause."

This shows the importance of hygiene in that area. That is why some dermatologists claim that poor hygiene is the most common cause of pruritus ani. After defecation few persons clean this area properly. In many Eastern countries pruritus ani is scarcely known, because in these countries toilet paper is not used, but people wash after every bowel movement. It is best to get used to having a bowel movement the first thing after arising, followed by a bath. Colored toilet paper should never be used, nor soap, since, says a famous dermatologist, this might introduce a further irritant.

In concluding this section, may I say that allergies can be cleared up by the right diet, the taking of the necessary food supplements and vitamins, and exercise.

I cannot speak too highly of exercise, especially walking, and in walking, choose the most precipitous hills. It takes from 5 to 10 times the energy to negotiate a steep hill compared to walking on the flat . . . which is almost a waste of time to inveterate walkers.

Go into training physically and the terrors of pruritus ani will vanish into thin air, provided you help along with diet, such as no sugar, salt, refined foods, etc. It is as simple as that.

Pruritus ani is most common in persons who lead a sedentary life and who eat the common American refined diet, including lots of orange and grapefruit juice.

CHAPTER 5.

NUTRITIONAL PREVENTION

Thus far we have taken up the subjects of foods that cause itching. We have discussed general causes of itching and pruritus ani (itching rectum). Now we shall deal with nutritional methods of *preventing* pruritus. That good nutrition is a definite preventive of conditions that cause itching, is generally recognized in medical literature.

Dr. Robert Turell, in *Surgery, Gynecology and Obstetrics* (104: 233, 1957), says in reference to treating pruritus ani, "Food intake should be well balanced and abundant in *all* vitamins, particularly the vitamin B complex. Tea, coffee, excessive carbohydrates, highly seasoned foods, and alcoholic beverages are to be avoided."

N. Philip Norman, M.D., in *The New International Clinics,* vol. 4, series 4, 1941, says, "True pruritus ani is caused by faulty, or improper nutrition. The prolonged subsistence upon a faulty, or improper diet causes a disorganization of the biologic processes (enzymic, microbic, excretory, secretory, etc.) of the intestinal tract. The protective function of the intestinal mucosa is impaired and bacterial infection occurs to complicate the condition. At this point, some form of nutritive failure becomes manifest, due to the inability of the digestive tract properly to digest and absorb nutritive essentials, many of which are either absent, or present in minimal or subminimal amounts in the faulty diet.

"The results obtained in a series of 38 cases of true pruritus ani, upon a co-operative basis, in which constructive dietetics was the major therapeutic factor, strongly supports the hypothesis that pruritus ani is a secondary or indirect expression of improper nutrition, and the direct expression of a fundamental disturbance of the physiologic function of the intestinal flora."

That pruritus ani is due to an improper diet is true in my own case. Years ago I used to get it from overeating citrus. Today, after years of strengthening my body with very good nutrition, I have tested it, by eating oranges and grapefruit daily, but there was no pruritus in the anus.

A physician writes to the editor of *The Journal of the American Medical Association* (Aug. 9, 1958), asking for the best method for treating intense rectal itching caused after long-time use of antibiotics. The editor replies that ultimately relief usually comes if the use of antibiotics is shunned. Then he states, "Adequate intake of vitamins and vitamin supplements should be stressed."

A lack of vitamin B in the body is directly associated with conditions of itching. Burning soles of the feet are known to be caused by a lack of the riboflavin portion of the B complex. This can be murderous in its intensity, and it is amazing how it clears up when the deficiency of this vitamin is corrected.

Dr. I. Dainow, of Geneva, Switzerland (*Dermatologia*, 92: 25-29, 1946) obtained sensational results in curing all kinds of pruritus with 17 patients who were treated with pantothenic acid and nicotinic acid (niacin) both part of the vitamin B complex. Dr. Dainow feels that the cures were effected through the antihistamine actions of these two vitamins.

Drs. Sisi and Plas-Arditti, in the *Semaine Hôpital* (Paris), January 20, 1954, issue, point out the frequent existence of pruritus localized at the anus and thereabouts with very burning sensations, as complications of antibiotic treatment, especially aureomycin. These prurituses, they say, seem to be caused essentially by the awakening of fungus infections and by deficiencies in vitamin B, which cause a destruction of the normal intestinal flora. These doctors suggest a course of the complex B Vitamins plus such things as yogurt and whey to permit the normal intestinal fibers to re-establish themselves.

Dr. W. Ray Shannon, M.D., writing in *The Urologic and Cutaneous Review* (December, 1942) states, "During the past winter I stumbled upon the fact that fantastic doses of thiamin chloride could control the painful itching of chilblain." Thiamin chloride is another of the vitamin B complex. Dr. Shannon obtained relief from itching by using this vitamin in chilblains, measles, hives (urticaria) eczema, itching skin, chicken pox, poison ivy, scabies, itching ears and pityriasis rosea. The latter is a skin condition characterized by eruptions on the back, legs, arms and thighs. Dr. Shannon states in review that "out of 35 cases, 22 or slightly more than 62% were entirely relieved of their itching within a phenomenally short time after treatment was started. Less than 18% could be called total failures. Those remaining (7 cases) were improved sufficiently to be considered as successful by the intimate observers. This method of treatment could thus be considered as worthwhile in somewhat more than 82% of the cases in this series . . . The doses were tremendous in terms of accepted daily requirements of this vitamin."

There are many other medical researches that reveal how helpful the administration of various parts of the vitamin B complex is in cases of pruritus. It would seem, therefore, that if a person made sure that he took an extra daily dose of vitamin B (brewer's yeast, wheat germ and desiccated liver) he would insure himself against the development of pruritus.

Now let us see the part vitamin A plays in this condition. In a case of pityriasis (described above), as related in *The Lancet* for September 18, 1954, p. 591, when the "patient was given large quantities of vitamin A, the pityriasis subsided notably and the area of induced lichenification also improved despite continued scratching. But this returned to its former intensity when the vitamin was discontinued."

Dr. J. Ferreira-Marques, in *The Archives fur Dermatologie and Syphilis* (Bd. 197, 85, 1953) states that in handling 40 cases of pruritus ani vitamin A was the medicine of choice. He believes that pruritus ani is caused by an abnormal secretion which irritates the nerve endings of the anus. Vitamin A normalizes the metabolism of the glands surrounding the anus and in so doing causes the itching to disappear.

We could cite many other cases where vitamin A was effective in reducing the pruritus but we had better get on to vitamin C and its place in curbing conditions of itching. In *The British Medical Journal* of February 13, 1954, page 366, there is the statement, "The nutritional disorders due to deficiencies of iron, vitamin A, vitamin B_2 group, vitamin C, and other essential elements, may lead to a loose hyperkeratosis (the enlargement of an organ, or part of one, due to an increase in the size of its cells), with a degree of atrophy (wasting away in the size of tissue) causing discomfort and an itching skin."

In an experiment written up in *The Archives of Dermatology and Syphilology* (February, 1954), 145 patients with various kinds of pruritus were treated with procaine hydrochloride alone, and in combination with vitamin C. The combination including the vitamin C showed much better results than the drug alone.

Vitamin C is the skin vitamin, a lack of it contributing to scurvy. A lack of vitamin C causes the skin to bruise easily. When the body has sufficient vitamin C, the skin is usually strong and healthy and will resist rupturing due to itching and scratching.

My young son years ago was very susceptible to poison ivy, but one year when we were on a no-bread diet, he was not bothered at all with it. When he was eating bread, he did not have the room or appetite for vegetables which are rich in vitamin C. On the vegetable diet his skin became healthier and did not become inflamed from the poison ivy sap or fumes.

Vitamin E has been used with success in connection with itching of the female organs at change of life. M. F. Block, M.D., writing in *Clinical Medicine* (60: 1, 1953), treated 10 patients with this condition and obtained excellent results with 8 of them. Vitamin E has the effect of oxygenating all tissues everywhere in the body, including the skin.

Calcium is another element that is of extreme importance in the health of the skin and in preventing the occurrence of itching. W. T. Kruse, M.D., writing in *The Journal of the Michigan State Medical Society* (Nov., 1952), describes an experiment with 26 patients with various kinds of pruritus coming from eczema, hives, etc. The patients were given calcium by mouth and also in a calcium-containing ointment that was applied to the affected parts, 80% of the patients reported excellent relief.

In this respect the use of white sugar in the diet causes a reduction in the body's calcium content and should be avoided if one is susceptible to pruritus. I once knew of a case of psoriasis which required terrible bouts of scratching. It was kept in check with vitamins, and the girl was warned against the use of sugar. But once in a while she weakened, and the pruritus always flared up again because of such lapses.

Hives are a condition commonly associated with an allergy to foods, especially to strawberries, but also to nuts, berries, shellfish, fresh fruits (especially the citrus), eggs, chocolate and pork. Sometimes the condition is more chronic and is due to foods eaten daily such as cereals, milk, vegetables, meat, etc. In more than half the cases emotional causes are suspected. But as with other forms of pruritus and allergies, a fortification of the body with good nutrition is the best preventive.

This is also true of prickly heat, which leads to violent itching and scratching. Dr. Robert L. Stern, reporting in *The Journal of the American Medical Association* (January 20, 1951), describes how vitamin C was given to troops in the South Pacific Islands during World War II and brought relief in a half hour. Similar results were obtained in Coachella, California, which is on the edge of a desert. So if you want to prepare yourself for hot weather, increase your dosage of rose hip vitamin C.

Sometimes prickly heat is induced by the taking of salt tablets. In tropical Karachi, at the R.A.F. General Hospital, during the last war it was noted that patients who got prickly heat had been taking extra salt, in the belief it was replacing salt lost in perspiration.

I heard from a doctor once that prickly heat is sometimes caused by a period of profuse sweating after the winter . . . during which time the body seldom perspires.

The sudden perspiration irritates the sweat glands in some way. After a week or so of warm weather, the glands become acclimated and the condition disappears.

I believe that the eating of sunflower seeds makes for a healthy skin. I have noticed this in my own case. In a controlled experiment with our chickens at our farm, one group had sunflower seeds added to their ration. Their feathers developed a finer sheen than the control birds. Seeds are full of vegetable oils that contain polyunsaturated fatty acids. In the Institute for Metabolic Research, at Oakland, California, there was the case of a 42 year old woman who, among other things, was suffering from a severe generalized pruritus. Part of the treatment was the taking of polyunsaturated fatty acids (ethyl linoleate and safflower oil). There was a dramatic and sustained fall in her cholesterol. The pruritus became less intense. Had she also been given the proper vitamins, I am sure there would have been a complete remission of her itching symptoms.

For a healthy skin eat all kinds of seeds —sunflower, pumpkin, peas, nuts, etc.

Seeds, eaten raw, are full of life-giving substances which can make for healthy tissues all over the body, including the skin.

What we have been telling you sounds almost like the whole *Prevention* System—the taking of vitamins A, B, C and E, calcium (bone meal), no sugar, and anything else that contributes to bodily health will contribute to skin health. Nutrition is the first defense when pruritus shows its ugly head.

Chapter 6.

SCABIES

In the consideration of the question of itching or pruritus we must include scabies, although in polite circles it is rarely seen these days. Even in the lower income groups the general availability of bathing facilities has greatly reduced this scourge. But where populations are low in personal hygiene it is still to be found. Sometimes it is brought in by carriers, as happened recently in an epidemic of it in several wards of a hospital. It is to be seen where people are crowded in barracks or in dormitories, and during wartime it flares up.

The scabies must not be confused with lice, cooties, or "crabs" which are an entirely different order of nuisance. Scabies are caused by a minute parasite or insect called *Sarcoptes scabici,* which can barely be seen with the naked eye. It has been referred to as the "Seven Years Itch," because careless people do not check it the easy way using sulphur ointments. They pick at the mites with their fingernails, desperately hoping to eliminate them, and only succeeding in becoming permanent hosts to the little pests. The mites burrow into the skin, some of the burrows being as long as a quarter of an inch. Sometimes they show little black dots which represent their excrement. The females lay eggs in the burrows, while the males wander over the surface of the skin, not venturing too far away from the family burrow.

In an average case of scabies, there are about 50 to 500 of the mites, but cases have been seen consisting of up to two millions of them.

They infest the hands, wrists, feet, buttocks, elbows, penis and scrotum, armpits and breasts. They can be "caught" from toilet seats, public towels, on door-knobs or umbrella handles, sleeping in a bed recently occupied by a carrier, etc. In 90% of the cases the affliction is transmitted by direct personal contact . . . a shake of the hands, for example. Anyone who has suffered from the actions of this parasite knows how excruciating their itch can be, causing raw abrasion of the skin by scratching. Yet they can be controlled very easily and quickly. Sulphur ointment P.P. has been found to be 97 to 100% effective.

This condition should not be confused with swimmer's itch found in the region of the Great Lakes. It is caused by flukes that burrow into the skin. These flukes live in the tissues of common snails. Bathers are infected by them from drops of water which are not wiped off the skin after bathing. The body should be dried immediately upon emergence from the water. Once in the skin they are destroyed by the body's defense forces, but a local irritation remains for a while at each point of entry. There is a decided itching.

A case was described in *The Journal of the American Medical Association* (June 7, 1958) in which a woman suffered from a severe pruritus caused by mites. The cause was finally discovered to come from bird mites. There was a window air-conditioner in which there were some bird nests, the birds evidently being infested with these mites. But before the correct diagnosis had been made, the woman had been called a neurotic because of her scratching.

One doctor has stated that 80% of night scratchers have worms of some kind—one of the most common being threadworms which attack in the genital regions and in the rectum. In a study in Washington, D.C., 41% of whites were found infested with them, but only 16% of the Negroes. This is fortunate because so many Negroes handle food in restaurants. This condition is extremely contagious. Some physicians blame it on our modern way of living. A Dr. E. C. Faust blames the wearing of underpants which generate heat in the genital region.

These worms are not microscopic. The female is 1/6 to 1/2 of an inch long . . . the males somewhat less. The worms live in the caecum, appendix and nearby points in the intestine, from which the females go to the rectum to deposit eggs. A female worm can lay an incredible number of eggs—up to 20,000.

Infection comes from hand-to-mouth, from the air inhaled from contaminated bedclothes or garments, from infected towels, soap, on floors, upholstery, etc. In one square foot of a large dining room 119 eggs were found, in a small classroom 305, in a toilet, 5,000.

The whole family must undergo treatment if the threadworm is to be completely eradicated. I will not discuss the drugs advocated. It is best to see a physician if one is infected with threadworms.

For the above information on the threadworm I depended mostly on an article in *The Irish Journal of Medical Science* by Dr. Ethna MacCarthy (Feb., 1951).

No discussion of scabies is complete without consideration of the itch that harrassed Napoleon for most of his days. Forty thousand books have been written about The Little Corporal. Fortunately one of them is completely devoted to the emperor's itch and is called *The Emperor's Itch*. It is by Reuben Friedman, M.D. (Froben Press, New York, N.Y.).

In the book he quotes Erasmus Wilson: "James the First, a royal authority, is said to have remarked that the itch was fitted only for kings, the scratching being so exquisite an enjoyment." According to Dr. Friedman, some of Napoleon's biographers believed that his itch almost cost him his life. Napoleon died of cancer of the stomach at the age of 51, but suffered from the itch for his entire adult life.

We know the typical picture of Napoleon with the fingers of his right hand inserted within his waistcoat. There have been various theories advanced for the mannerism. Some have called it merely a mannerism, others say it was due to gastric distress. Some have attributed it to eczema and a desire to scratch, while still others think it was due to the itching of scabies that he tried to relieve.

Boris Sokoloff in his *Napoleon, A Doctor's Biography*, says "Throughout the years of his rise to power, Napoleon suffered from a skin disease which he had acquired at Toulon. Replacing a slain cannoneer at his post, he became infected with the disease then rampant throughout the French army. *La gale,* a scabby skin infection was jestingly called *la gratelle* (the scratch), or more endearingly, *la charmante*. 'Everyone was scratching,' remarked an observer, speaking of the army in Italy. Whole regiments of soldiers, the moment they were encamped for the night, threw off their knapsacks and scratched en masse."

Dr. Cabanès in *Journal des Maladies cutanees et syphilitiques* 4: 411, 1892, wrote: "It was at the siege of Toulon, in 1793, that Napoleon, who was then only a colonel in the artillery, contracted scabies under circumstances which have not, perhaps, been accurately reported. A cannoneer had just been killed at his station. Colonel Bonaparte, seeing the battery thus out of commission, took a ramrod in his hand and loaded the gun himself several times. A few days later the emperor's entire body presented an eruption having all the characteristics of scabies. . . .

"Popular belief accepted the legend of scabies as true. Indeed some one even composed a quatrain on the subject, which passed from mouth to mouth:

"One day Napoleon took me by the hand,
A favor without equal

Saying, 'Tomorrow you will have
something from me'
And the next day I had scabies."

Napoleon probably did get the scabies at this time, but Cabanès says he was cured of it by taking sulphur baths and other treatments. The itch that he suffered for so many years must have been something else, for his hygiene habits were flawless. He was known to spend hours daily in his bath.

Here is a quotation cited by Dr. Friedman from Wayne Whipple's *The Story of Napoleon*. "All his life Napoleon was hampered and tantalized by an itching 'humor' in his blood. In boyhood it took the form of hives, which irritated him and made him nervous, frantic and ungovernable. At maturity it came out a skin eruption which his enemies called the itch (scabies). When it did not show itself on the surface it acted like a strange fire within. The physicians called it *pruritus*, and it seemed to fill his mind with an abnormal pruriency, exciting him to passions insatiate, unknown to normal man.

"This 'hell-fire within' humiliated and exasperated him in the keenest crises of his career. In the heat and struggle of a great battle his blood was warmed to such a maddening degree that, instead of being able to stay where he could superintend the conflict, he was found, under cover, stripped to the skin, lying on straw or on the bare ground, surrounded by his aides, who were scratching his quivering flesh till his blood flowed while he was shouting at them: 'Harder! Harder! As if you were currying a donkey!'. . . . This blood tincture was hereditary. It reproduced the malignant internal cancer of which he died, as did his father and grandfathers, for many generations. . . . It must have been pathetic to see the ghastly inroads the pruritus had made upon his ambition. That internal cancer seemed to be devouring his very soul."

There can be no doubt that if Napoleon had scabies it was something that came and went. The itch which remained with him had other causes. This is shown by the following from Cabanès: "During the Egyptian campaign, (1798-1799), Napoleon, having suffered several gastric attacks (he was already experiencing the first symptoms of cancer, from which he finally died), was covered with clothes worn by a scabietic in order to bring back the eruption." It was believed in those days that the eruption of scabies was helpful in driving off certain toxic elements from the body.

Another proof that Napoleon's condition was not scabies is the fact that his wife Josephine never had it. Desclaux stated, "Would it not be more logical to think that this pruritic skin condition of Napoleon was the prurigo of Hebra, an affection which is common among people with arthritis." According to *The American Illustrated Medical Dictionary*, prurigo is a "chronic skin disease marked by the development of small, pale papules and intense itching. The papules are deep-seated, and the disease begins in childhood and lasts through life, being usually incurable."

After discussing a few other possibilities upon which he throws cold water, Dr. Friedman offers the theory that Napoleon was suffering from *dermatitis herpetiformis* (Duhring's disease), a rare disease in which there is intense itching and burning, and the cause of which is unknown. Sometimes it has been confused with eczema. If I may be so bold, I would like to conjecture that dermatitis herpetiformis may have an emotional origin, in Napoleon's case caused by the tensions of war and battles and the torments and petty badgering of his political administrators. It also might strike at persons who are vitamin and mineral deficient.

Dr. Friedman refers to a case of dermatitis herpetiformis described in *The American Journal of the Medical Sciences* (January, 1885). "The patient, Capt. K., 34 years old, of previous good health and normal skin, while gunning in the meadows, almost lost his life by suddenly sinking into a bog, from which after a half-hour's struggling he at last succeeded in extricating himself. Three days later he developed dermatitis herpetiformis and thereafter remained subject to recurrent attacks of it. 'I am still troubled with the disease,' wrote the patient to Dr. Duhring,

4 years after he had first seen him."

Napoleon was still afflicted with his itching on the island of St. Helena and "told Dr. Antommarchi, his personal physician on the island, that his itch was of regular occurrence, and dated from the siege of Toulon." Evidently something must have happened at Toulon which was a severe blow from an emotional standpoint, because it was from that time that he was possessed of the itch on a permanent basis. Dr. Friedman indicates that under the psycho-therapeutic management of Dr. Corvisart, "in whom Napoleon had complete confidence, its symptoms rapidly abated, but he was never really permanently free of pruritic crises."

Finally, Dr. Friedman states that Napoleon's characteristic pose was probably merely a mannerism, cultivated since boyhood.

I would like to reproduce a portion of Dr. Friedman's appendix called *La Galle,* from a book *Album Comique de pathologie pittoresque,* published by Ambroise Fordieu, 1823.

"Uncleanliness is one of the most active causes of the itch. That is why it so furiously attacked those Russian troops whose pestilential odor is still remembered in France to this day. The suffocating vapor that accompanied, preceded and followed them for long distances was so intense that, in the famous campaign of Friedland, it was even made use of successfully by our experienced generals. The approach of the Russian columns was scented by them at a distance of one or two leagues. Indeed, sensitive noses detected them even at three leagues. As a matter of fact, a number of our officers were deployed for no other than reconnaisance purposes. The Russians, advancing in great number, betrayed the secrets of their movements and positions by their odor. Whenever the question was heard in the Frank ranks: 'Do you smell anything on the left?' it was sure to be the right wing of the Russians. And when our ranks cried out: 'Phew! What a stench!', it was almost always the center of the muscovite phalanxes."

Chapter 7.

ARE DRUGS THE ANSWER?

The Wall Street Journal, in a very comprehensive article about drug firms and itch remedies, says, "Medical researchers have conquered at least half a dozen dread diseases in the last 10 years, but they are still largely in the dark, they admit, in finding relief for one age-old ailment—the itch . . . Drug executives foresee a market of $35 million a year for potions and pills that would do away with the annoyance of the itch. Doctors estimate that as many as 20 million to 30 million people in the U.S. come down with some form of this affliction every year."

One drug firm struck a right note when it said recently that its product works by removing the desire to scratch, but that it would be better to eliminate the cause of the itch. The salves and ointments are only palliatives. A physician says that doctors are pretty much in agreement that most drug store medicines are worse than none at all. "In the majority of cases," he said, "these ointments and lotions are too harsh. Literally, they add insult to injury. As a matter of fact, in at least half of the cases of itching the causative factor is not a skin disease but a general medical problem."

Another physician: "During the past 5 years (before 1955), at least 60 different new preparations have been reported to be of aid in the treatment of pruritus (itch). Almost all of these have not been adequately controlled, and in the future will probably be relegated to obscurity, like so many medications of the past."

A doctor refers to the usual treatment for the itch as being wholly empiric. Empiric means experimental, based on experience, rather than by reasoning or theory. But at best it is a case of guessing, or trial . . . and error.

When the patient becomes frantic with itching one authority gives reserpine and chlorpromazine, both high-powered tranquilizing drugs. They calm the patient and make it easier for him to bear the itching.

This, according to the authority, gives the doctor a chance to focus his attention on "treating" the skin trouble, but rarely to remove the cause.

A local anesthetic type of salve called dyclonine gave relief in most of 200 cases of itching, but some of them reported irritation and other signs of sensitivity. I wouldn't want to take this drug because it might just be my luck to be sensitive to it.

Another anesthetic type of drug for the itch is procaine and it is advised to be taken either by mouth, injected into the veins, or applied on the itching skin. One would be foolish to swallow this stuff for an inch when there are sensible ways to go about discovering and eliminating the cause of it. Incidentally, a medical article says that procaine is about one-fourth as toxic as cocaine.

How does procaine act? "It affects all living cells, but its main action is on the nerve fibers, where it produces an attenuation in the condition of impulses." In other words, the effect is to fool you, to get you to stick your head in the ground. The itch is still there but it is kept from your nerves, which would ordinarily dispatch the message to your brain, telling you that you itch, and that you should begin scratching. For my money, I'll take prevention. This article says, "A patient highly sensitive to procaine will develop untoward symptoms within a few moments after its use." And they reassure us that they "were unable to find any report of fatality, due to the oral administration of procaine. But some of the symptoms resulting from oral administration were headache, dizziness, weakness, nervousness, nausea, drowsiness, flushing, heartburn, vomiting, fatigue, cramps, diarrhea, abdominal pain, frequency (of urination?), belching, visual disturbance, and palpitation. No, thank you. Not for my money.

Here is another statement from a different journal: "In general, cortisone, hydrocortisone, and ACTH given systemically tend to relieve itching, but these are powerful drugs, and if the underlying cause of the pruritus is not removed, then prolonged administration is necessary, with its subsequent dangers."

There are Burrow's solution, camomile extract, Lassar's paste, amino acid ointments, amphetamine, methyltestarone, injections of alcohol, and tattooing of the involved skin with mercuric chloride in the case of pruritus vulva (the female organs), and a thousand other drugs and procedures.

But the use of ointments can be dangerous to the interior of the body. One imagines that they remain only on the surface of the skin. But that is not so. They can be absorbed into the blood stream. Take a case reported in the *Archives of Dermatology and Syphilology* (29: 382, 1934). A dentist aged 52 suffered from a pruritic condition diagnosed as scabies, and a sulfur ointment was used on 6 successive days, applied over his entire body, including the face. The condition became much worse. He had had a normal heart condition. He became very uncomfortable. His entire skin became brownish red, and he was given colloidal tub baths with various soothing remedies. He went from bad to worse and died of acute interstitial myocarditis within a few days. Myocarditis is an inflammation of the muscular walls of the heart. Interstitial pertains to the interstices or interspaces of a tissue.

According to this article, this type of myocardial failure often comes after ointments are used on some skin conditions. Cases are mentioned such as a man with an infected burn, a carbuncle on the neck, an abrasion of the arm, a skin infection of the groin, etc. A typical case was an infection of the foot that was treated. Thirteen days later there developed cardiac (heart) symptoms.

The article winds up with the following statement. "It seems timely to emphasize the disastrous results that may follow the indiscriminate use of proprietary remedies."

In an article in the *Journal of the American Medical Association* (157: 720, 1955) the problem of the overtreatment of skin conditions is stressed. Many of these remedies produce other skin diseases which the author terms "overtreatment dermatitis," and the users "drugstore physicians." One hundred and fifty thousand such cases are reported annually. L. E.

Gaul, M.D., the author of the article, says that the statistics show that overtreatment dermatitis is in the top quarter of common skin diseases in the country.

When it was first announced that sulfonamides could be used in skin ointments, the incidence of overtreatment dermatitis increased greatly. But soon reports began to appear like that of the A.M.A. Council on Pharmacy and Chemistry which warned of the dangers following the external use of the sulfonamides. Reports like this seldom get much attention in the newspapers, so, although doctors knew of the warnings, the general public went right ahead rubbing the sulfa preparation into their skins, and overtreatment was the final result.

Turning to local anesthetics, antihistamines and topical antibiotics, we find the same results. Local anesthetics reverse their intended effect, that is, instead of relieving itching, they cause it.

I found an advertisement of one drug product that is worth mentioning. This is Borcherdt's Malt Soup Extract, for use in cases of pruritus ani (rectum). A Dr.

Louis H. Brooks is quoted in the advertisement as saying: "It was found that administration of Malt Soup Extract in dosages of one or two tablespoonfuls twice daily produced favorable results. Within two or three days after beginning this simple regimen, the itching and burning usually disappeared." The advertisement claims that the malt extract works by restoring the normal acid condition in the lower tract and by promoting the growth and development of aciduric bacteria. Whether this does the job or not, at least the malt extract is a rather bland substance and cannot do much harm.

In closing, I present a letter sent by a physician to the editor of the *Journal of the Australian Medical Association* (June 28, 1958). He speaks of a case of pruritus vulvae. The vulva is the near-the-surface part of the organs of generation of the female:

"Dear Editor: As a medical student I eagerly frequented the houses of dermatologists and physicians in Macquarie Street and there was prescribed for with a frankness that drove from my heart the young and magic mystery of medicine. For my advisers would read the textbooks with me and between us we would pick a seeming-good prescription. And so, with the years, the pruritus continued on its own way and my patients derived some ever temporary benefit from my own sufferings and from the ointment and lotion sections of the various hospital pharmacopoeias and the dermatology books. Finally, I became convinced I was one of the great living experts on pruritus therapy. That was till I met my first case of pruritus vulvae in my then country practice. The red, swollen and irritable vulva appalled me, but I assured the lady she was being advised by a specialist—and the cocaine and its congeners, the carbolic and the calamine, the hygiene, the rest and all the sedatives drove my patient to a dermatologist in Brisbane, and lo! to my surprise and chagrin (?), she was back in her country home in two weeks bright and cured, except, of course, for the little itch that is the pleasant reminder. The specialist was kind enough to let me have his secret: 3% silver nitrate dissolved in nitrous spirits of ether—which I soon got going onto myself. Oh! the piquant agony of the application; the fiery apnoeic, psyche-consuming, nerve-tingling half-minute. Then the glow! and then the ease! Paradise for days! With ensuing applications, ease for months; then forever—but ever with the remnant occasional prod to recall the intense rawness of other days.

"So my patients and I developed a technique—and they were keen to use the doctor's personal treatment—the 'silver ease.' Wash with cotton wool and soft soap and water after defaecation. Clean underwear daily. Bath twice daily. No greases or lotions. Apply the nitrate solution with a soft brush—liberally—with the nates well spread. There is time for this swift liberal application before the silver burn arrests all activities. Finish off by applying a layer of witch-hazel vanishing cream—which seems to smooth off skin roughness and at least has a delicious cooling sensation. No more silver is applied till the pruritus again drives you to it.

"Any man who treats himself has a fool for a doctor—and if so, in this case we can agree with Pope:

You think me cruel? Take it for a rule,
No creature smarts so little as a fool.

"Or with Ausonius:

Mules may ease each other's itch.

"Dr. Wilson, and you, sir, will, I trust, detect no hint in all this that pruritus ani may be associated with 'pruritus disputandi.' "

June 2, 1958.

Yours, etc.
H.O.T.

Chapter 8.

RELIEF WITHOUT DRUGS

May I present a few letters from readers who have suggestions to offer in regard to the control of itching? E. H. McElyea of Long Beach, California, wrote us as follows:

"*Prevention* readers might like to reap the benefits of my painful, expensive experience with an itching rectum—pruritis—from which I suffered twenty years.

"I was informed by a large hospital staff where they treat only the rectum and colon that this was a nerve disease which could be cured only by surgery. They cut a slit about three inches long, one and a fourth inches deep front to back through the opening, then cut several small places around the opening, and cut the skin from the flesh to kill the nerves. They were almost successful in killing the nerves, as I was unable to control my bowels for two years and am not entirely over it after nine years. The itching stopped for about eight months, then it came back as bad as ever.

"Yes, they guarantee the work. All I had to do was go back and go through the torture again. There would have been no charges other than medicine, dressings, room, board, etc. This possibly would have cost about $150.00. However, I did not go back.

"After some time, I located a doctor who said I had a stubborn case, but that if I would follow his instructions to the letter he would straighten me out. Following are his instructions:

"I must at all times have cotton, Witch Hazel, Vaseline, gentian violet, Desenex Ointment, a rubber glove or finger cot, and corn starch. Before elimination, put on the finger cot and lubricate the passage with vaseline. After elimination, wash with water using cotton. Dry with cotton, apply gentian violet, allow to dry, and then apply cornstarch. The Desenex Ointment may be applied instead of the gentian violet from time to time as desired.

"Three calls at his office and material

purchased added up to a total of $35.00. I still use cotton and corn starch after elimination, and if I feel any irritation, I sterilize with Witch Hazel. No one can clean himself thoroughly without washing."

It is possible that this man's pruritus might have been cured by a process of elimination in connection with what he was eating. It could have been an over-consumption of orange juice. There have been complete and permanent cures merely by the elimination of this juice from the diet.

T. D. Somerville of Plymouth, North Carolina, in connection with itching in the rectum and especially that caused by hemorrhoids, says, "I have found and advised many of the care of this itching and the forming of projections on the rectum, and have been told that it really works on many mild cases as well as on some bad ones. The oil on one's hands and fingers is one of the best oils to kill bacteria and this same oil has a great healing power over the tender flesh of the rectum. With a bit of Vicks, Mentholatum or Vaseline to lubricate, and with a clean hand or fingers that have not been washed for a few hours, as on arising in the morning, a gentle massage will in a few days relieve this pain. However, it is not a complete cure.

"The animal family also gets sore and itchy and Nature has told them and built them in a way to take care of themselves. Nature gave this same care to man, if he would only use it. This trouble could be greatly reduced in the human race."

Here again, there can be no question that hemorrhoids are of nutritional origin —that is, they are caused by the use of foods that are not completely digested, and the residues of which are irritating to the outgoing passages or contain strong acids. Foods that are rarely completely digested are products made of wheat and rye, such as bread, cereals, spaghetti, etc. Sufferers from hemorrhoids would do well to eliminate all grain foods.

Grant Jeynes, whose place of residence will not be mentioned, says, "On two occasions my pruritus ani became so bad I had to see a doctor. Witch Hazel I have found to be wonderful for this trouble. In my case (this was a third occasion last spring) occasional application of Witch Hazel stopped the itch in two weeks and I've not had it since. Besides, I find it possible to eat things such as sunflower seeds, citrus fruits, etc., which before were causing trouble."

This is the second time I heard that sunflower seeds could produce an itch. But almost any food could do it to some individuals who happen to be allergic to that food. In the case of sunflower seeds, I believe that those allergic individuals might be able to tolerate a small amount of them. They are too valuable an item of food to be completely eliminated from one's diet.

It is interesting to note that this man finally could eat citrus fruits without getting pruritus. I have found in my own case that my increasing health, due to better nutrition and to exercise, etc., has also eliminated many food allergies for me.

Here is another experience with pruritus ani that comes from "A *Prevention* reader," who lives in Minneapolis, Minnesota. "This condition I have had since

1952, and no doctor seemed to be able to help me. Five weeks ago I started to take a salt water enema every other day (one tablespoon of salt to a quart of water) and it appears I've got it licked. You may print this or not, as you see fit. If it helps only one person of all your readers, I think you have done a great service to mankind."

Salt is a strong substance. For an occasional use it may be all right. But I would not recommend it to be included in enemas that are taken regularly. In fact, I would not recommend the regular taking of enemas, although there are many who swear by them.

Veering away from pruritus ani, Mrs. C. E. Wilson of Rittman, Ohio, says, "Red clover teas is sure to cure hives."

Sister Veronica, of a Sacred Heart Hospital somewhere on the Pacific Coast, writes: "I read with much pleasure and profit *The Healthy Hunzas*. I congratulate you and wish that book were read by everybody. (Note: It had a very poor sale for some reason.) But the purpose of my letter is this: In this book you mention a girl who, on the advice of a woman doctor, ate raw potatoes and was thus cured of eczema. We had a case of eczema here. We tried raw potatoes with great success."

For those who cannot stomach whole raw potatoes, they could cut into small pieces and mix with fruit in a Waring Blender. This would be a splendid dish and at the same time extremely healthful.

Now on to the subject of how to treat itching without drugs.

Dr. Rolf Ulrich in his book *Coffee and Caffeine*, says that in an experiment with eczema cases who were given coffee, all reported that they felt warmer and that the affected part itched worse than before and showed a redness.

It is a known fact that pruritus is aggravated by heat. A physician states that itching is increased by the vasodilating effect of heat and decreased by cold. He states, however, that if the heat sensation is sufficiently intense, the resulting burning might abolish the itch. Vasodilation means the enlargement of the blood vessels. This in the case of the application of heat, causes an inflammation.

One method is to diminish the symptom by replacing it with something else. Baths or soaks can accomplish this, or even the application of water with with wash rags, preferably cool water. This doctor suggests putting starch in the water. He also suggests the application of calamine lotion.

Cooling the skin is one of the best ways to give relief. The cold dulls the nerves and produces an anemia in the skin. Menthol has also been used for this purpose, but it is only temporary in its relief. However, I would like to caution you against running cold water on the feet. They are a dangerously vulnerable spot for cold water. If you have to put cold water on them, follow it immediately with hot, alternating cold with hot.

Perspiring is one of the causes of pruritus. That is why it is desirable for an obese person to reduce, for the excess weight brings on excess perspiration. Such a person sweats heavily between the legs causing a pruritus there. Perspiration is healthy but after a period of perspiring one should wash it off the body. Recently

I had an itch between the legs. I used to bathe once a day. But when I washed 3 times a day I got it under control more or less . . . once in the morning after a night of perspiring—once after my daily walk in which I merely sit in the tub with water only covering the pruritic area, and again the same position in the tub before going to bed. If it is not convenient to use 3 tub baths, one can use a wash rag or sponge.

To prevent too much perspiration one should use the minimum of bed clothes and, if necessary, employ an electric heating device in winter under the bed sheets. One should wear loose underwear and clothes that are not too tight. I found in my case that I frequently sat in a narrow chair with side arms that kept my feet too close together, and this caused much perspiration in the midsection.

Cleanliness is of the greatest importance, especially in pruritus ani and in women in pruritus vulvae which involves the sexual area. There must be cleaning after each urination and bowel movement and in doing this there should be patting, not rubbing, with soft toilet paper, cotton or tissue. One should not scratch. One physician advises, "Scratching only aggravates the itching, and much greater relief can be obtained by pinching the portion of skin that itches or by applying firm continuous pressure on the involved parts with the closed fist or fingers."

A dry itching skin is another cause of pruritus, especially in people in the 50's and 60's. Sometimes it is referred to as senile pruritus. A panel of dermatologists at Columbia University recommended a mixture of 10% olive oil, 70% lanolin and 20% water, applied directly to the skin to eliminate such dryness.

A Dr. Rein of the above-mentioned panel, advises that showers be discontinued by persons suffering the itching skin that is so bothersome to many people in winter especially. He tells us that colloidal baths can be valuable in softening and lubricating scaly and itchy skin. Such a bath can be made up in this way: a cup of oatmeal is put in a container with two teaspoons of oil (olive, corn, cottonseed or peanut oil), mixed with a quart of milk, then poured into a tub of lukewarm water.

The patient then soaks himself in this solution. The soothing warmth of the water, coupled with the fats and oils, is intended to restore softness and moisture to the skin. Greasing the skin with more of the same type of oil is recommended after the bath.

The entire panel of dermatologists was unanimous in its condemnation of the use of soap. They agreed that the skin is only irritated by the chemicals contained in soap, and each time it is used it introduces new dryness and itching to the skin. The panel also recommended that one avoid rubbing with a towel, but rather that one pat the skin dry, thus preserving the oils and avoiding added irritation.

One physician has found that a change of climate was very effective. Harold Eidinoff, M.D., reporting in the *Journal of Investigative Dermatology,* followed the record of 34 cases of intractable pruritus of various kinds who were living in a low-level, humid climate area. "When these patients left the low humid climate and moved to a high dry climate, all but 3 of the 34 were able to achieve a practically complete remission or improvement, some within a relatively short time. This was accomplished without any other treatment by some patients," while most of them had the effect of exposure of the parts to the natural sun. These patients went to El Paso, Texas.

Dr. Eidinoff goes on, "The patients who recovered remained generally well (except for occasional minor relapses) as long as they stayed in the high dry climate. A return to a low humid climate for any length of time often resulted in a severe recurrence of the disease. By returning to a high dry climate the dermatosis again cleared, except in one case.

The climate condition of El Paso is altitude 3,700 feet, average temperature 70 degrees F. Average humidity 35%, rainfall 10 inches per year. The effect of a high, dry climate is to increase the rate of water evaporation from the skin.

Last year I had an itch in the midsection and was able to get it nicely under control, but when we went to Palm Beach for the entire winter, it came back. This section of Florida is a low-level, high humidity area and should be shunned by sufferers from any kind of pruritus. They should favor certain sections of Texas, Arizona, etc. What a lot of scratching must be going on in such places as Palm Beach, Miami, etc.!

Chapter 9.

SKIN PROBLEMS ON CONTACT

The dialing of a telephone results in a ring of blisters around one victim's index finger; another finds that turning his car key and zipping his brief case have caused the itchy blisters that are so bothersome. The patient suffers from contact dermatitis, or, more simply, skin disease from the touch of an object. In recent years, tracking down the cause of dermatitis conditions has become highly specialized, and sometimes the search may go on for months. Success depends on many factors, including the ingenuity of the doctor in interpreting the shape and type of skin disturbance as well as the patient's powers of recall. The doctor must puzzle out, from just where the sores appear and how they develop, what object one would contact only in these spots, and whether it is liquid or solid, round or flat, rod or rope, etc. Then, to cooperate, the patient must try to record his every contact throughout the day, he must try to remember any changes that might have occurred in his daily schedule—any clue he can offer might carry in it the key to his problem. Imagine, of the thousands of things one touches in a day, narrowing the suspects down to the dial of a telephone! This dermatology business is tricky.

We are told in Dr. George Waldbott's book, *Contact Dermatitis* (published by Charles C Thomas, Springfield, Ill.), that all age group are subject to contact dermatitis. Even infants of a few weeks of age have been known to be sensitive to their mother's lipstick. Incidence is shown, however, to be more prevalent in later life than in the early years. Also, women are known to be more susceptible than men—the percentage of women who suffer from contact dermatitis is almost double that of men. Though it has not been proven, it is supposed that the large variety of cosmetics, hair dyes and perfumes employed by women account for this difference.

The normal skin has built-in defenses against the invasion of foreign elements.

These are two important barriers, the horny layer of epidermis and the oily secretion of the sebaceous glands. Substances which are capable of destroying either of these defenses are those which are most likely to reach the living cells beneath the skin in sufficient quantities to cause sensitivity which shows itself in the form of itchy or painful blistering and scabbing.

The materials which are most likely to penetrate the skin or usually oily in character—plant oils or certain lubricating oils cling to the fatty covering of the skin and dissolve more readily than water soluble materials. Certain dyes have the ability to become fixed in the horny layer of the skin. During their prolonged stay, the elements of the dyes come into intimate contact with the sensitive cells, and eruption of tiny blisters often results. Other common offenders are metallic salts and local anesthetics.

All of these sources are easily contacted in an ordinary day's activities. The plants which give off oils which cause dermatitis are common enough, ivy, oak, sumac, chrysanthemums, ragweed, certain bulbs, etc. The dyes are everywhere: leather shoes, wallets, belts, colored clothing, furs, gloves and many more objects that are dyed, including soaps, fingernail polishes, hair rinses, toilet tissues, powders and lipsticks. Among the metals nickel and aluminum are the worst offenders, but can one get through a day without contacting one of these somewhere in his normal activities?

Perhaps it is well here to discuss more specific causes of dermatitis which can and should be avoided in anticipation of the trouble they can cause. Chief among these is cosmetics. The general use of cosmetic products among women and men in the United States has boomed the sales to well over a billion and a half dollars per year. And some of these are actually dangerous in every sense of the word!

Hair dyes, for example, contain metallic salts, such as lead, copper, silver and iron, as well as anilin dyes which are especially harmful. Even the vegetable dyes used in these preparations (henna, indigo and walnut) contain damaging components. Infections are not uncommon and even death from the use of hair dyes has been reported in extremely sensitive cases.

Dr. Waldbott warns that no one should permit her hair to be dyed without careful preliminary testing. Even if the dye has been used before without ill effects, subsequent applications might still be dangerous since the skin could have become sensitized in the interim. We say, stay away from hair dye entirely. It makes the hair coarse and robs it of any body and resiliency it might possess. Besides, nothing is more attractive than hair, no matter what its color, which is kept well-brushed and neatly arranged, and which is healthy due to proper nutrition. The health-minded person will always avoid hair dye of any kind.

One of the questions which keeps recurring in our mail is this: How can one get clean without using soap? Critics of our stand against the use of soap will be interested in the opinion of Dr. Waldbott, one of the country's outstanding allergists, concerning this matter: "A patient can take his daily baths without soaps and cleanse his body sufficiently by gently rubbing the skin with a dry towel after the bath." It is well known that soaps can cause dermatitis in sensitive persons, and in those not so sensitive, who are frequently exposed. Further, the use of soap is likely to aggravate any existing skin problem no matter what its original cause. Sensitivity to soap is usually attributed to coloring matter, or the medications and perfumes included in various kinds. But the basic composition of soap makes it a natural troublemaker. The soap molecule includes an oil soluble fatty acid and a water soluble alkali. The alkali softens and dissolves the protective layers of the skin, and both it and the fatty acid are likely to produce skin irritation. Since we know that soap isn't essential in cleansing the body, why invite the problems of soap dermatitis by using it?

You can pick up a dandy skin problem from the use of drugs too. Dr. Waldbott tells us that, "Any allergic disease as well as practically every known dermatological break in the skin may result from sensitivity to drugs." There is no drug whatsoever that is free from sensitizing properties. These two facts alone should serve as sufficient caution against the indiscriminate use of drugs. And remember, aspirin is a drug; pep pills and tranquilizers are drugs. Avoid them. Substitute good diet for them, and you'll soon see a pleasing difference in yourself.

Dr. Waldbott brought out an interesting point in his book with regard to food sensitivity. He says that contact with the food itself is not always the cause of a reaction, but the disinfectants and insect sprays that are on it might be. Not to be forgotten are the toxic colorings on citrus fruits, and those chemicals used in wrapping and packaging the food (e.g., colored papers, plastics) for they often contain sensitizing agents.

Consider the possibilities of contact dermatitis in daily life, and try to avoid having possible causes of this uncomfortable disease around you. Avoid cosmetics especially for they are great offenders. Above all, keep your nutrition at a good level, for a healthy body can minimize the effects of harsh irritants to the skin.

Chapter 10.

PSORIASIS CAN BE HELPED

Every day there are men and women throughout the country who look in the mirror and discover little red patches that weren't there before on their elbows and knees. The patches are covered by white or yellowish scales. If they are scratched, the scales become silvery and flake off like dandruff. Sometimes the red patches itch, sometimes not. But they are unsightly, and their name has become synonymous with embarrassment. These men and women have discovered on their bodies the unpleasant disease called psoriasis.

If you spot these symptoms, and you go to your doctor, you might be disappointed by his treatment. The medical profession has acknowledged no definite cause for this unsightly disease, and no sure cure. Your doctor may recommend some combination of salves, ointments and compresses to give you short term relief. Hopefully, however, he will investigate your diet.

Research indicates that psoriasis is at least partially a disease involving defective metabolism, and fed by a faulty diet. Of those experimenters who have treated the disease with any measure of success, many have concerned themselves chiefly with the elements of diet involved in fat metabolism.

Doctors Paul Gross and Beatrice M. Kesten from the Department of Dermatology at the Columbia-Presbyterian Medical Center, reported success in treating psoriasis with soybean lecithin in the *New York State Journal of Medicine* (Vol. 50, 1950).

The doctors eliminated eggs, fat meats, poultry, fish, cheese and excessive amounts of butter and cream from their patients' diets in order to run the experiment on a strict low-fat regimen. The lecithin was distributed to the 235 subjects, along with vitamins A and D and the B vitamins thiamin, pyridoxine, riboflavin and pantothenic acid. Because of the restricted diet, the doctors considered it important to administer vitamin supplements, but are certain it was the lecithin that was responsible for the therapeutic value in this case. Out of the total figure, 155 patients were considered adequately treated. The rest either did not cooperate or abandoned the diet before any conclusions could be drawn.

The results of the experiment were encouraging to psoriasis sufferers. Twenty-three of the patients remained well after one year of therapy and three years of observation. Only 37 patients experienced no improvement. Of the remaining people, 29 were satisfied with the way their psoriasis was being controlled. The other 66 subjects showed some improvement, but required therapeutic ointments in addition to the lecithin in order to bolster their progress.

Doctors Gross and Kesten concluded that, "this form of therapy is capable of correcting some of the metabolic defects but not the actual cause of the disease." They recommend a low-fat diet and the addition of a lipotropic, or fat-emulsifying substance such as lecithin to control psoriasis, "just as proper diet and supportive treatment alone can control many cases of diabetes."

Other medical experimenters have praised lecithin in controlling psoriasis. An article in *Your Health* (Fall, 1949) entitled, "New Hope for Psoriasis," describes a new medicine which had been successfully tried on a small number of patients. The article, written by Herman Goodman, M.D., one of the country's best-known dermatologists, describes the medicine as "one of a group of lipids—fatlike chemicals— which include lecithin and vitamin A." The body needs lecithin, which is rich in unsaturated fatty acids, other important fats and the B vitamins, in order to use fats properly.

Eczema in children has been known to disappear almost miraculously when fats containing lecithin or the unsaturated fatty acids were added to the diets of children. In fact, Adelle Davis, in her book, *Let's Eat Right to Keep Fit* (Harcourt, Brace and World, New York), says, "Even the stubborn eczema-like condition known as psoriasis usually disappears rapidly when salad oils and lecithin are added to the diet."

Faulty diet and defective metabolism may lead to psoriasis. But the relationship doesn't stop there. The skin disease may drain your body of essential nutrients and create a further deficiency in your body.

In 1965, Daphne Roe, M.D., a dermatologist and nutritionist at Cornell University, told the annual meeting of the New York State Medical Society that psoriasis may be more serious than is usually assumed. She warned that the constant loss of skin tissue can cause enormous losses of vitamin and mineral nutrients. Even people who eat a normally good diet may develop nutritional deficiencies in the wake of this disease.

At the same time Dr. Roe proposed dietary means to control this supposedly incurable disease. She and her affiliates at Cornell had already successfully stopped psoriasis through diet.

According to Dr. Roe, studies at the Clinical Nutrition Unit of Cornell University have shown that psoriasis comes about because of a metabolic defect, probably in enzyme production, that renders the body unable to handle normally the amino acid, taurine. Taurine is not one of the essential amino acids. It is formed within our own bodies. But apparently our bodies rarely, if ever, manufacture enough taurine to do any great damage, even if it cannot be handled.

It is the excess of taurine that we obtain from the foods we eat that causes psoriasis, if we lack the metabolic ability to use it properly. The ultimate and convincing demonstration of this is that the people at Cornell have successfully gotten rid of psoriasis in a group of patients and kept those patients rid of it for periods up to two years with a diet that was deliberately low in taurine.

This is not exactly a cure, but is rather what the doctors call a control. That is, the patient is cured as long as he sticks to his special diet. If he should return to consuming large amounts of taurine, the psoriasis would probably return. It is generally true of metabolic defects, of which diabetes is the most prominent example, that they cannot be cured, but can be controlled indefinitely.

Control of taurine intake, however, is not quite as simple as insulin control of diabetes. Practically all proteins, from porterhouse steak to herring, contain substantial amounts of taurine. As Dr. Roe pointed out, protein is an absolutely essential food and you cannot dispense with it just to eliminate the taurine it contains.

Fortunately, the Cornell experimenters found another method. They discovered that taurine is extremely susceptible to leaching in boiling water. By insisting that their patients boil all meats for at least five minutes, and throw away the cooking water before broiling, roasting or whatever else they intended to do with the food, they managed to eliminate the major part of the taurine contained in these meats.

This is not a cooking method that we would recommend to anybody who is not suffering from psoriasis. In terms of flavor and texture, boiling is usually the worst thing you can do to a piece of meat. In nutritive terms, it is absolutely sinful. It will remove all the water-soluble vitamins, which means the entire B complex and whatever vitamin C there may be in the food. It will also leach out important minerals.

No, we do not recommend boiling meat or indeed any food, except for this special purpose of controlling psoriasis. If you have psoriasis and must do this, then there is another obvious step you must take. That is to be sure of taking vitamin supplements, which were as important a part of the Cornell therapy as the low-taurine diet.

In stressing the problem of finding a protein food with low taurine content, Dr. Roe said that such foods were being developed, and pointed out that soybean products "seem promising."

If you are bothered by psoriasis it really becomes necessary to be conscious of every mouthful of food that you eat. Avoid meat and dairy fats. The only fats you eat should be those containing lecithin—eggs, salad oils and fats from other vegetable sources such as sunflower seeds, avocados and raw nuts are healthful fats.

Eat your meats, poultry and fish broiled or roasted, without gravy. Eat plenty of fruits and vegetables, as many as possible raw. Ignore desserts, except for raw fruits. Sugar and white flour rob your body of B vitamins.

Baker's bread (any kind of bread made in a factory) may contain a variety of unhealthful fats, even including synthetic ones made of chemicals with no relation to food at all.

Make certain you are getting among your food supplements enough vitamins A and D (plentiful in fish liver oils), and the B vitamins (wheat germ, brewer's yeast or desiccated liver are your best sources), lecithin and/or the unsaturated fatty acids available in flakes or in capsules.

Lecithin supplements, derived chiefly from soybeans, should be a staple in the diet of every psoriasis sufferer. (Whole soybeans are also rich in calcium, iron, other trace minerals, and the B vitamins and vitamin E.) If you hope to control or avoid psoriasis, keep an ample amount of soybeans or soybean lecithin in your diet.

CHAPTER 11.

VITAMIN A FOR SKIN DISEASES

For many long years the patient with psoriasis has suffered in silence, scratched in private and, when the lesions were particularly bad, isolated himself from the public gaze. Psoriasis does not shorten life, the dermatologists maintain, though sometimes its victims wish it would.

The victim of psoriasis is caught in a most unhappy bind. His disease is one which through the ages has baffled the skin doctor and defied his ingenuity. "Psoriasis is an antidote for the dermatologist's ego," P. Bechet, an eminent dermatologist and medical historian once remarked. The pesky scaling disease drives its victim to try everything in the dermatologist's medicine bag—tar, mercury Chrysarobin, phenol. Some of them do bring a measure of relief. Then—boom! The eruptions are back in full bloom, bigger than ever, redder, itchier and more repulsive. He has probably tried x-ray therapy, which too can bring dangerous relapses, warns John Goodwin Downing, M.D., professor of dermatology, emeritus, Boston University and Tufts University Schools of Medicine. (*The New England Journal of Medicine,* June 11, 1959)

Indications are, however, that soon the victims of psoriasis can throw away their dangerous drugs and begin to really live. Our old friend, vitamin A, is again making medical headlines as a substance which, in its acid form, can relieve the ugly blotches of this pesky skin disorder. This was determined by Phillip Frost, M.D., and Gerald D. Weinstein, M.D., of the Department of Dermatology, University of Miami School of Medicine. In a double-blind controlled study they found that vitamin A, in its acid form, did indeed bring remarkable relief from the itching and unsightliness of psoriasis in 24 out of 26 patients. These effects were noticeable after only one week of treatment. (*Journal of the American Medical Association,* March 10, 1969)

Before they undertook a clinical study

of vitamin A acid, Dr. Frost and Dr. Weinstein first compared the effects of several commonly available forms of topically administered vitamin A on three patients with extensive psoriasis and three patients with lamellar ichthyosis (dry, rough, scaly skin). They used four pieces of cotton gauze on afflicted areas on the arms of each patient, and covered each piece with adhesive tape. Then they injected a solution of vitamin A acid, vitamin A aldehyde, vitamin A alcohol, and vitamin A acetate through the tape into the square pieces of cotton gauze which were in contact with the skin.

After 48 hours, when the patches were removed, they noted slight softening of the skin in all the patch areas. They marked the patch sites and observed them daily. After one week, the area which had vitamin A acid applied to it showed markedly decreased scaling in the patients with the dry rough scaling skin of ichthyosis and much less erythema (redness caused by congestion of the capillaries) in those patients with psoriasis. No changes were discernible where the other forms of vitamin A had been applied.

Intrigued by the superior healing properties demonstrated by this simple patch test, Frost and Weinstein then began a more extensive evaluation of vitamin A acid.

They chose patients with some ugly skin conditions that are most resistant to all kinds of treatment—10 with epidermolytic hyperkeratosis, in which the skin becomes hard and loose; 24 with some form of ichthyosis and 26 with extensive psoriasis. Control bases containing no vitamin A acid were applied to an involved area on on side of the patient's body, and a preparation that looked exactly the same but which contained either .1%, .2% or .3% vitamin A acid, was applied to an area on the other side of the body that was comparably involved. Preparations were coded in a double-blind fashion, so that neither patient nor physician was aware of which side would receive the "active" mixture.

What were the results? Vitamin A acid

scored major points in almost every patient, especially those with disorders which do not usually respond to the dermatologist's efforts. While both sides of the patient's body showed improvement when the affliction was a mild form of ichthyosis, in no case did greater improvement occur on the control side.

The improvement was dramatic in those patients with psoriasis. The side treated with vitamin A acid showed a decrease in scaling and redness in 24 out of 26 patients, and improvement was evident in as little as one week. (Most improvement was shown after 3 weeks of treatment.) Nine out of the patients showed a complete clearing of the side treated with vitamin A acid and no improvement on the other side. Eleven showed a moderate improvement, and four showed slight improvement.

Frost and Weinstein point out that, to be effective, the vitamin A acid solution should be either a .2% or .3% concentration. When German investigator von Beer used a .1% vitamin A acid preparation on 20 patients, there was no noticeable improvement. The Florida investigators believe their more favorable response is due to the use of the higher concentrations.

It is interesting to note that the improvement resulting from vitamin A acid usually lasted 10 to 14 days after discontinuing therapy. After this period, both control and active ingredient-treated sides began to look similar.

As Frost and Weinstein point out, the clinical use of vitamin A was originally based on the observation that in certain laboratory animals and in humans, vitamin A deficiency was associated with scaling of the skin. This cleared when vitamin A was added to the diet. It may be, though it has not been proven, that the person with psoriasis has an inordinate need for vitamin A. He should certainly get the maximum safe dosage.

Halibut liver oil is an excellent source of both vitamin A and its working partner, vitamin D, which might also have an ameliorative effect on psoriasis. D is the sunshine vitamin and it has been observed that psoriasis improves in the summer because of exposure to the sun. It almost never appears on the face and hands because these areas are exposed to the sun more than the rest of the body.

Physicians have given 200,000 units daily for six months, according to J. M. Lewis *et al.*, writing in the *Journal of Pediatrics* (31, 496, 1947), without observing any signs of toxicity. We would not recommend more than 50,000 units of vitamin A daily, however, unless you are being supervised by a physician. It is not generally known, but years ago it was determined that what sometimes seems to be a deficiency of vitamin A, is actually a deficiency of vitamin E. Unless vitamin E is amply supplied, the vitamin A obtained from both foods and supplements, the vitamin A already in the blood, and that which is stored in the liver and other body tissues, is quickly destroyed by oxygen. (*Biochemical Journal*, 34, 1321, 1940)

If you have psoriasis, you would do well to double the usual requirements of the mineral supplements—bone meal and dolomite tablets. The same holds true for all the vitamins. Put special emphasis on vitamin C as found in rose hips and wheat germ for the B-complex vitamins.

Vitamin F or unsaturated fatty acids has been found to be about 25 to 50 per cent lower in the blood of psoriasis patients than in healthy persons. Dr. Sigwald Bommer gave a wheat germ oil preparation to one patient who was completely cured within a few weeks of a stubborn case of psoriasis, which for many years had resisted all treatment. Other patients on the wheat germ oil showed some improvement. (*Munich Medical Weekly*, Vol. 26, p. 1308, 1961)

The fact that the symptoms of psoriasis are in part similar to those of arthritis, and that the two diseases are sometimes found associated, prompt the suggestion from John J. Miller, Ph.D., in the *Journal of Applied Nutrition* (Dec., 1964), that arthritis may aggravate psoriasis and vice versa. Therefore experience would indicate that vitamins A, B-complex, D, A and E would be beneficial, it was pointed out by C. Reppert *et al.* in *Proc. Soc. Exp. Biol. Med.* (77, p. 318-1951).

It has been found that carbohydrate metabolism is faulty in psoriasis. This indicates a heightened need for both magnesium and zinc, says C. H. Beck in *Dermatologica* (vol. 104, p. 171, 1952). And since it has long been known that thyroid tends to normalize the utilization of cholesterol by the human body, magnesium and the B-complex vitamins are again indicated, Dr. Miller says.

If you are suffering the tortures of the ailment which has thus far defied the dermatologist's skill, try to improve your nutrition. Eliminate processed foods that are loaded with saturated fats. Increase your supplements and you may find that your health and outlook and skin will improve to the point that you won't need the vitamin A acid when it becomes available. It's worth a try.

Chapter 12.

ITCHY FEET? IT COULD BE ALLERGY

Shoe contact dermatitis, once a medical curiosity, can no longer be considered rare, according to Dr. Ernst Epstein, of the Division of Dermatology of the University of California, San Francisco Medical Center. Writing in the *Journal of the American Medical Association* (September 8, 1969), Dr. Epstein says that in the past three decades allergy to shoes has become much more common. He reports on 74 suspected cases seen at his Medical Center over a five year period; in the case of 43 the skin disorders were found definitely caused by shoe allergy, and allergy "probably or possibly" caused the dermatitis in the case of nine others.

The material in shoes that most frequently triggers allergic reaction is found in the rubber-based adhesives used universally in by shoe manufacturers in this country, according to Dr. Epstein. The rubber is processed by various chemicals, and it is these substances that usually do the damage. Other compounds have also been implicated to a lesser extent—dyes, coal tar resins in the adhesives, and chromates used in tanning the leather, for example.

He and his colleagues found that nearly half of their patients had been using antifungal remedies prior to coming to the Medical Center. Either they or their physicians, Dr. Epstein says, held the mistaken belief that they were dealing with the fungal infection, athlete's foot.

Antifungal remedies are not only ineffective in treating an allergic disorder. They actually make matters worse. Often the person who has allergic sensitivity to shoes is also sensitive to the ingredients in the medication. The rash becomes further irritated, the skin breaks, and pus sometimes forms.

If you have skin trouble on your feet, how can you tell if you should suspect that you are allergic to your shoes?

In its typical form, Dr. Epstein tells us, shoe contact dermatitis is quite distinctive. Characteristically, the rash appears on the tops of the toes and adjacent surfaces of the foot. The big toe is most frequently involved. The spaces between the toes, and the underportion of the toes—areas usually involved in athlete's foot—are typically unaffected when the dermatitis is caused by allergy. The soles of the feet also rarely show the allergic rash.

So if you have shoe dermatitis in its typical form, undoubtedly you will suspect at once after reading this description.

Unfortunately, many sufferers fail to conform to the typical. Dr. Epstein says that in about a third of the cases shoe dermatitis appears in one or more of all the uncharacteristic areas. It can show up on any part of the foot. So you have to look for other clues.

One unmistakable sign is a rash that exactly matches the portion of the shoe with which it has been in contact—for example, the strap of a woman's shoe. In such a case, you can be sure that you are allergic to those particular shoes and you should discard them at once.

Since the shoe's rubber-based adhesive is so often the allergen that produces shoe dermatitis, you might examine other areas of the body that have contact with rubber—elastic waistbands, for example. Is there any sign of a skin eruption there? If so, you have strong reason to believe that your foot condition too is due to sensitivity to rubber. Among Dr. Epstein's patients, several had waist dermatitis from underwear; a rubber garter strap had caused a rash on the thigh of one woman, and another had had dermatitis induced by a rubber bathing cap. In all these cases, the evidence of rubber-caused allergic reactions helped the doctors in their diagnosis.

Rubber allergy is not caused by rubber itself, but by the chemicals used in rubber processing. Fortunately, chemicals in the rubber-based adhesives vary. Thus you may very well be allergic to one pair of shoes and not another—even though rubber is present in both. Also, you may be allergic to the rubber in your shoes but not to the elastic band that holds up your underwear. So just because you *don't* have a waist dermatitis doesn't mean that you can discount the possibility of rubber-caused dermatitis on your feet.

Is it really necessary for shoe manufacturers to use known allergens in their products? Do they *have* to include material that will cause discomfort and pain to an unknown number of their clients?

The answer is no—they don't have to. There is actually one firm in the country that puts out a special product for people with allergy problems. This is the Derma Pedic shoe (made in men's models only) of the Brockton Shoe Company; the leather is vegetable-tanned (some people are allergic to aniline dyes), and a non-rubber adhesive is used. So we know that shoes *can* be made out of material that is safe for everyone.

The day may come when the government will be sufficiently concerned about consumer welfare to prohibit potentially harmful materials in the manufacture of shoes, wearing apparel and above all, food. Until then, like many other additive-caused allergies, shoe contact dermatitis will continue to be a problem to many. It can only be eliminated if it is recognized for what it is. We should all be alert to the possibility.